Your Healthy Whole Mouth

Book 2 of 12.

Learn the Lyrics of GarGar the Dentist's Song. Mouth Painting I Will Go

DR Garth D Pettit

Copyright © 2017 4 Your Smile 2 Shine Pty. Ltd.

All rights reserved.

ISBN: 13:978-1983617461
ISBN-10: 1983617466

DEDICATION

I dedicate this book to our daughter, Jacqueline.

Illustrations by Megan Spiers, of MeganSpiers.com

Model photos by Richard Coburn, Acoustics in Art.

DR Garth Pettit

Table of Contents

Visit 2 of 12 Visits to GarGar The Dentist

Learn the Lyrics of GarGar The Dentist's Song

Mouth Painting I Will Go

Sung toMelody of "A Hunting I Will Go"

Chapter 1: Introduction

Chapter 2: Notes

Chapter 3: Greetings From GarGar The Dentist

Chapter 4: Mouth Model Pictures

Chapter 5: Mouth Painting I Will Go Song Lyrics

Chapter 6: Author's eBooks

Chapter 7: Book Reviews, Websites , General Information

Book 2 of 12:: Your Healthy Whole Mouth.

Learn the Lyrics and Melody of GarGar the Dentist's Song Mouth Painting I will Go

DR Garth Pettit

Chapter 1

INTRODUCTION

How Do I Look After My Kids Teeth?

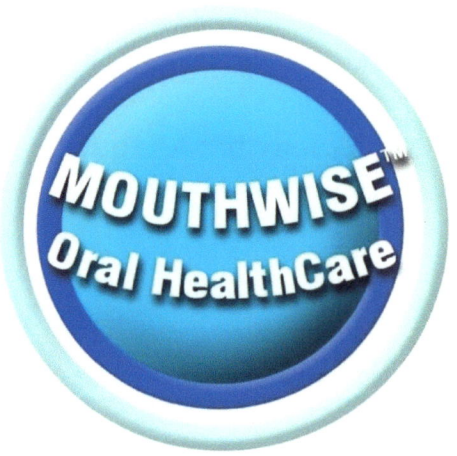

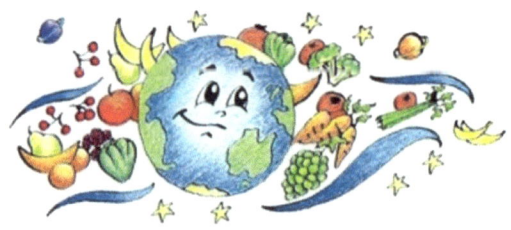

Book 2 of 12:: Your Healthy Whole Mouth.

Learn the Lyrics and Melody of GarGar the Dentist's Song Mouth Painting I will Go

DR Garth Pettit

My best advice in answer to the often asked question "How Do I Look After My Kids Teeth", or to any other similar or related questions, is summarized here:

Firstly: Give your children the best ever oral hygiene instructions that will predictably prevent common oral diseases such as tooth decay, gum diseases, bad breath, stained teeth and wrecked smiles. That instruction is Paint Your Mouth which is a 21st Century oral hygiene instruction. It is definitely not the instruction Brush Your Teeth which is a 15th Century tooth-only cleaning instruction.

Secondly: Give your children a simple, but thorough and comprehensive, oral health care education. An oral health care education that will educate your kids to become self-motivated to prevent oral diseases for the rest of their lives and to enjoy the lifetime benefits of an orally healthy mouth. That oral health care education is in this series of eBooks titled Teaching Oral Disease Prevention.

There is a total of 78 eBooks in this series of eBooks titled Teaching Oral Disease Prevention in Amazon.com. Although they are available in each of 6 editions: English, German, French, Italian, Spanish and Portuguese the foreign language translations are yet to be done. In each edition there are twelve individual, successive eBooks, 1 to 12 and one other eBook which includes all twelve individual eBooks. Details for each of these eBooks are listed at the end of each eBook.

Teaching Oral Disease Prevention eBooks are, without doubt, the most comprehensive, yet simple and ideal, children's oral health education eBooks that are available to anyone with any interest whatsoever in children's oral health care.

Book 2 of 12:: Your Healthy Whole Mouth.

Learn the Lyrics and Melody of GarGar the Dentist's Song Mouth Painting I will Go

DR Garth Pettit

My name is Dr Garth Pettit, I am an Oral Health Care Educator and Author and since 1996 I have been totally focused on this mission; *Prevent Oral Diseases In Children.*

Book 2 of 12:: Your Healthy Whole Mouth.

Learn the Lyrics and Melody of GarGar the Dentist's Song Mouth Painting I will Go

DR Garth Pettit

Chapter 2

Notes

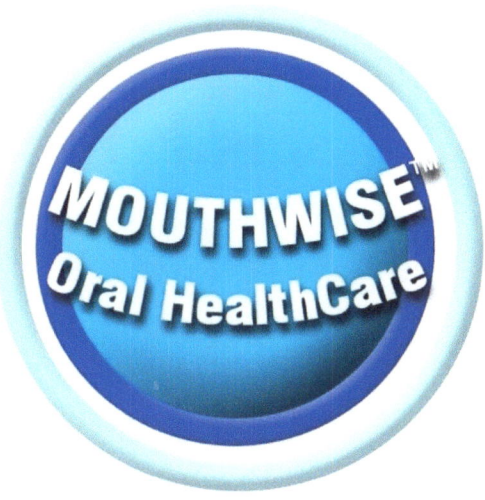

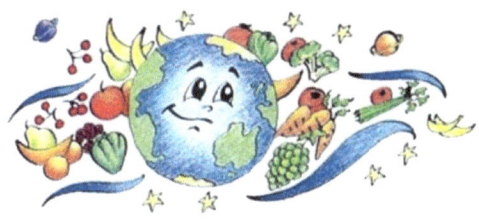

Book 2 of 12:: Your Healthy Whole Mouth.

Learn the Lyrics and Melody of GarGar the Dentist's Song Mouth Painting I will Go

DR Garth Pettit

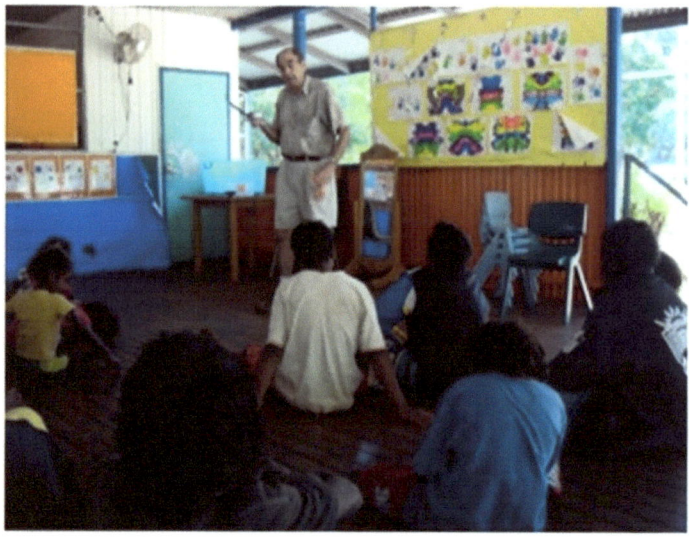

Graphic above: Author, Dr Garth Pettit teaching children, at a remote Aboriginal Community School in East Arnhem Land, Northern Territory, Australia, how to 'Paint Your Mouth'.

In fact it was taken on the day the author changed his Oral. Hygiene Instruction "Treat Your Whole Mouth (originally, in 2002, "Treat Your Mouth", early 2007) to "Paint Your Mouth" (late 2007). He asked them "would you like me to show you how to paint your mouth?" Their immediate, loud, spontaneous shouts of YES, YES, YES convinced the author to change his oral hygiene instruction to Paint Your Mouth.

Book 2 of 12:: Your Healthy Whole Mouth.

Learn the Lyrics and Melody of GarGar the Dentist's Song Mouth Painting I will Go

DR Garth Pettit

About The Author

After a 5-year retirement from dentistry the author returned to his profession in January 1997, with the specific mission 'To Prevent Oral Diseases in Children' by the creation of improved oral health educational resources. He chose to work in rural, Northern Territory of Australia, Government clinics to be closely associated with schools, parents, teachers and children.

To prevent oral diseases in children Dr Pettit believed it was necessary to educate children in a wide range of topics; oral health, oral healthcare (oral health care), oral disease, oral anatomy, oral disease prevention and most importantly in oral hygiene. He believed that children would become self- motivated to prevent oral diseases once they had been given a chance to learn and understand these subjects.

Dr Pettit finally retired from hands-on dentistry to concentrate on his mission: Prevent Oral Diseases in Children.

The original 10 books on which these revised eBook versions have been made were reviewed by The Education Departments of The Northern Territory of Australia and by The Education Department of Queensland, Australia. Both Education Departments recommended them for use in their schools.

Book 2 of 12:: Your Healthy Whole Mouth.

Learn the Lyrics and Melody of GarGar the Dentist's Song Mouth Painting I will Go

DR Garth Pettit

Chapter 3

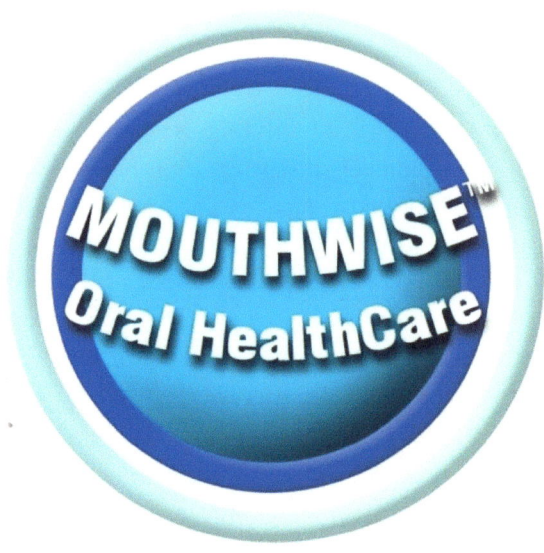

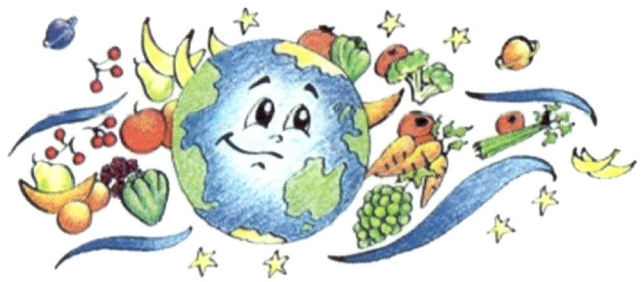

Book 2 of 12:: Your Healthy Whole Mouth.

Learn the Lyrics and Melody of GarGar the Dentist's Song Mouth Painting I will Go

DR Garth Pettit

Hi Kids, I Am GarGar The Dentist

That's me, GarGar The Dentist, on the right below and that's the real me, Dr Garth Pettit, on the left

To learn more about us you can search our names on the internet.

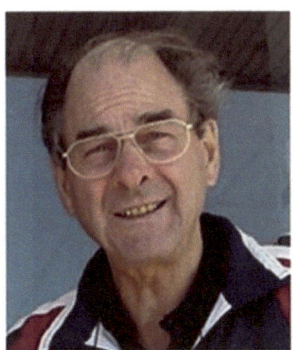

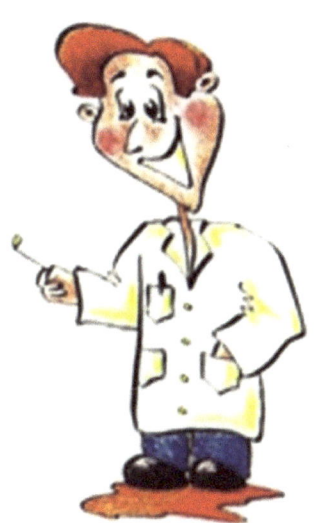

Book 2 of 12:: Your Healthy Whole Mouth.

Learn the Lyrics and Melody of GarGar the Dentist's Song Mouth Painting I will Go

DR Garth Pettit

I Warmly Welcome All Children in Our World

Preventing tooth decay, gum diseases, bad breath and stained teeth is simple if you know how. But statistics in 2017 confirm children still suffer from all of these easily preventable diseases.

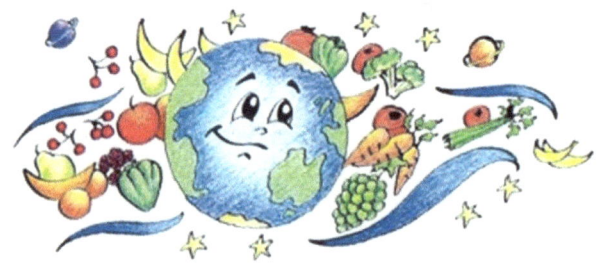

Kids, you sing this song, ♪ *Mouth Pain -ting I Will Go* ♪, to the melody of the nursey rhyme "A Hunting We Will Go"

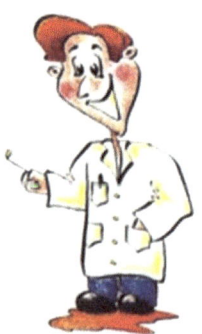

Book 2 of 12:: Your Healthy Whole Mouth.

Learn the Lyrics and Melody of GarGar the Dentist's Song Mouth Painting I will Go

DR Garth Pettit

Kids, 🎵 *Mouth Pain -ting I Will Go* 🎵 is another MouthWise Oral Healthcare fun song that will help you remember your MouthWise Oral 7 Hygiene instruction "Paint Your Mouth

It's easy to remember Oral 7 Hygiene because the 7 refers to All the things in your mouth.

Your mouth is like a house.

It has a roof, a floor, 2 side walls and a front door. It also has furniture; teeth, gums and tongue.

You will learn that each member of GarGar's SmileShine Gang represents one of the seven important surfaces inside your mouths.

So whenever you see their pictures you will know which surface GarGar is talking about.

But first, please study the pictures of the models in Part 2 to become familiar with the parts of your mouth before we go to GarGar The Dentist and the SmileShine Gang and the lyrics of 🎵 Mouth Pain –ting I Will Go 🎵.

Book 2 of 12:: Your Healthy Whole Mouth.

Learn the Lyrics and Melody of GarGar the Dentist's Song Mouth Painting I will Go

DR Garth Pettit

Chapter 4

Mouth Model Pictures

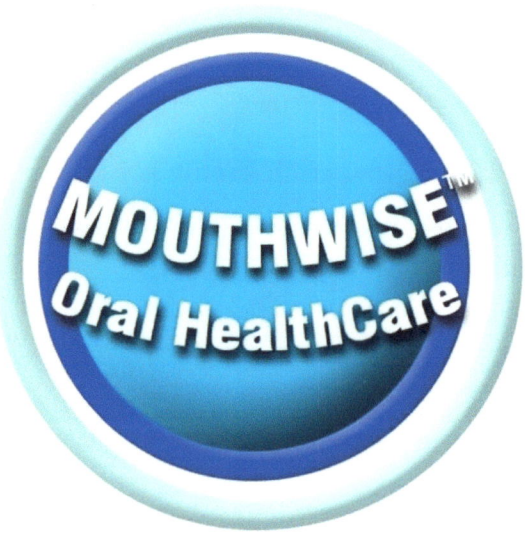

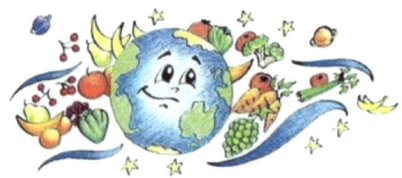

Book 2 of 12:: Your Healthy Whole Mouth.

Learn the Lyrics and Melody of GarGar the Dentist's Song Mouth Painting I will Go

DR Garth Pettit

These pictures will help you to learn some of the surfaces inside of your mouths that you will be painting.

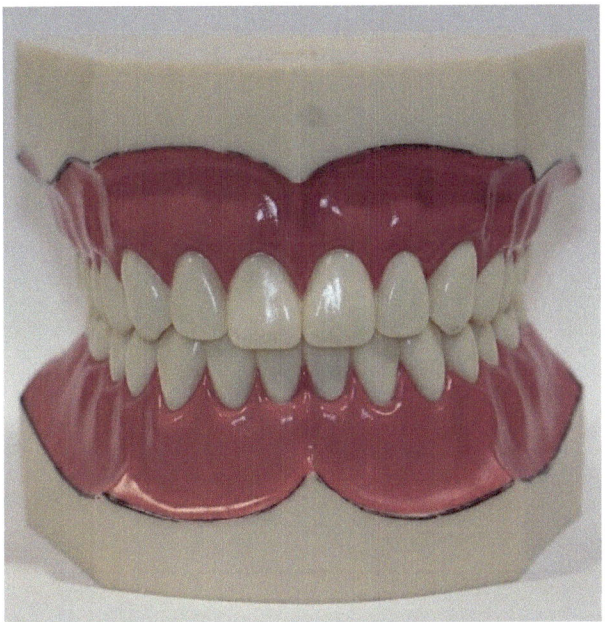

This model shows the outside surfaces of teeth and gums of your top jaw and your bottom jaw.

Please notice that the gum surfaces are ALL of the pink surfaces, NOT just the gum next to the teeth which is called the gingiva.

Book 2 of 12:: Your Healthy Whole Mouth.

Learn the Lyrics and Melody of GarGar the Dentist's Song Mouth Painting I will Go

DR Garth Pettit

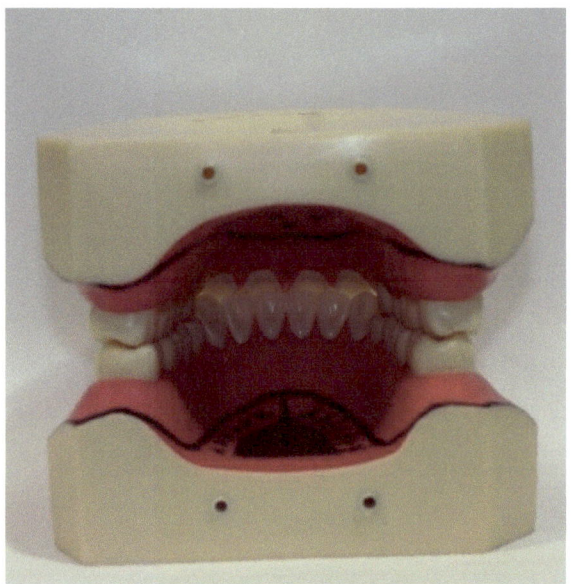

This model shows the inside surfaces of teeth and gums of your top jaw and your bottom jaw.

Please notice again that the gum surfaces are ALL of the pink surfaces, NOT just the gum next to the teeth which is called the gingival.

Notice the roof of your mouth in the top jaw and the floor of your mouth under the tongue in the bottom jaw.

Book 2 of 12:: Your Healthy Whole Mouth.

Learn the Lyrics and Melody of GarGar the Dentist's Song Mouth Painting I will Go

DR Garth Pettit

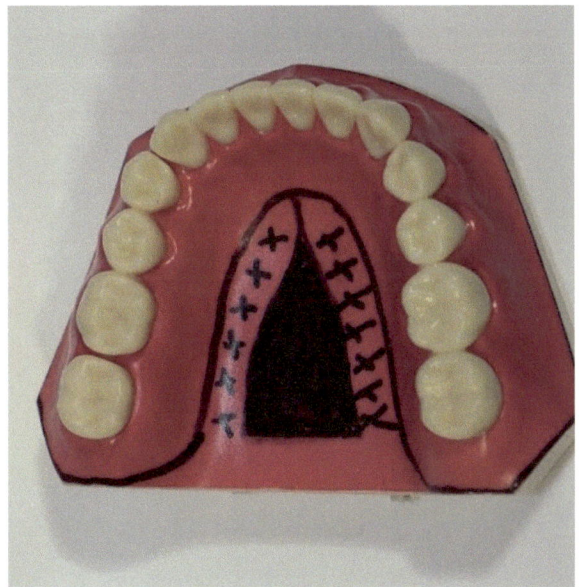

This model shows the floor of your mouth under your tongue more clearly where marked with crosses. The black area is where the tongue muscles attach to the floor.

It shows also the whole of your gums both inside and outside of the bottom jaw. And also the bottom teeth.

Book 2 of 12:: Your Healthy Whole Mouth.

Learn the Lyrics and Melody of GarGar the Dentist's Song Mouth Painting I will Go

DR Garth Pettit

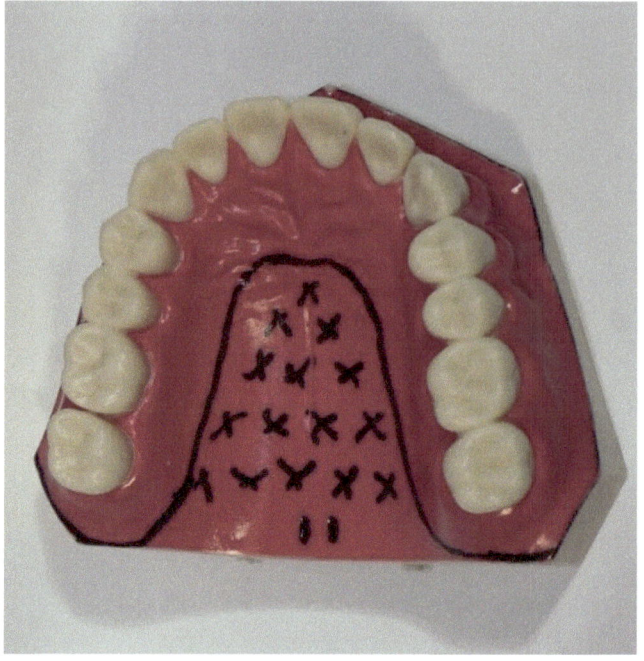

This model shows the roof of your mouth, the hard palate, more clearly where marked with crosses..

It shows also the whole of your gums inside of the top jaw from edge of teeth to the hard palate.

Also, of course, the top teeth and gingivae around the teeth.

Book 2 of 12:: Your Healthy Whole Mouth.

Learn the Lyrics and Melody of GarGar the Dentist's Song Mouth Painting I will Go

DR Garth Pettit

Chapter 5

Mouth Painting I Will Go Song Lyrics

Sung to the melody of the song "A Hunting We Will Go"

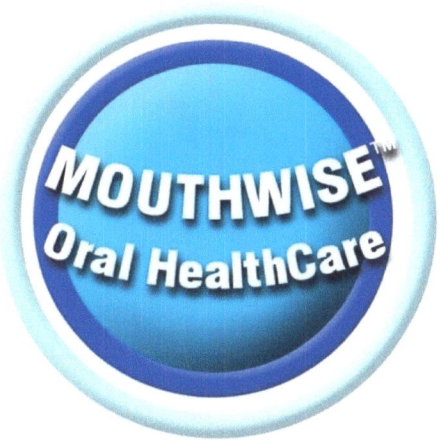

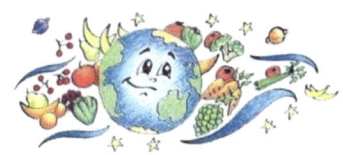

Book 2 of 12:: Your Healthy Whole Mouth.

Learn the Lyrics and Melody of GarGar the Dentist's Song Mouth Painting I will Go

DR Garth Pettit

♫ Mouth Pain –ting I Will Go ♫

Mouth   pain   -ting   I   will   go

Mouth   pain   -ting   I   will   go

I want a mouth   -wise mouth

Mouth   pain   -ting   I   will   go

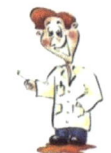

Mouth   pain   -ting   I   will   go

Mouth   pain   -ting   I   will   go

I want a heal   -thy   mouth

Mouth   pain   -ting   I   will   go

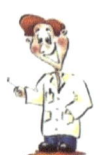

Book 2 of 12:: Your Healthy Whole Mouth.

Learn the Lyrics and Melody of GarGar the Dentist's Song Mouth Painting I will Go

DR Garth Pettit

Mouth pain -ting I will go

Mouth pain -ting I will go

I want a hap -py mouth

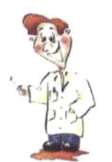

Mouth pain -ting I will go

It's fun it's fun it's fun

It's fun it's fun it's fun

I want a mouth wise mouth

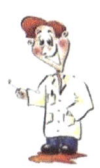

It's fun it's fun it's fun

I am so ex -cite -ted

I am so ex -cite -ted

I want a heal -thy mouth

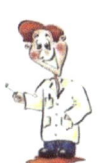

I am so ex -cite -ted

Book 2 of 12:: Your Healthy Whole Mouth.

Learn the Lyrics and Melody of GarGar the Dentist's Song Mouth Painting I will Go

DR Garth Pettit

Might jump o -ver the moon

Might jump o -ver the moon

I want a hap -py mouth

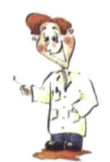

Might jump o -ver the moon

So here I go I go

So here I go I go

I want a mouth wise mouth

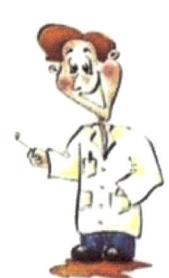

So here I go I go

Book 2 of 12:: Your Healthy Whole Mouth.

Learn the Lyrics and Melody of GarGar the Dentist's Song Mouth Painting I will Go

DR Garth Pettit

To   start   I   clean my   teeth

To   start   I   clean my   teeth

I want a   heal -thy   mouth

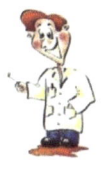 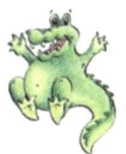

To   start I clean my teeth

And   then   I   clean my   gums

And   then   I   clean my   gums

I   want a   hap -py   mouth

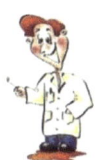

And   then   I clean my gums

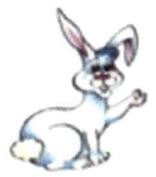

Book 2 of 12:: Your Healthy Whole Mouth.

Learn the Lyrics and Melody of GarGar the Dentist's Song Mouth Painting I will Go

DR Garth Pettit

I clean the top of tongue

I clean the top of tongue

I want a mouth wise mouth

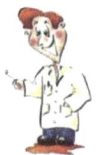

I clean the top of tongue

I clean floor un -der tongue

I clean floor un -der tongue

I want a heal thy mouth

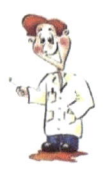 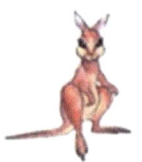

I clean floor un-der tongue

Book 2 of 12:: Your Healthy Whole Mouth.

Learn the Lyrics and Melody of GarGar the Dentist's Song Mouth Painting I will Go

DR Garth Pettit

And then I clean the roof

And then I clean the roof

I want a hap -py mouth

And then I clean the roof
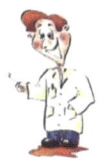

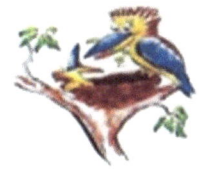

I clean in -side both cheeks

I clean in -side both cheeks

I want a mouth wise mouth
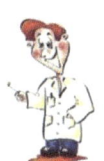

I clean in -side both cheeks

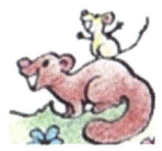

Book 2 of 12:: Your Healthy Whole Mouth.

Learn the Lyrics and Melody of GarGar the Dentist's Song Mouth Painting I will Go

DR Garth Pettit

    I   clean in -side both lips

    I   clean in -side both lips

  I want a heal -thy   mouth

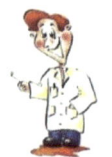 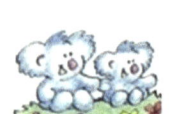

I   clean in -side both lips

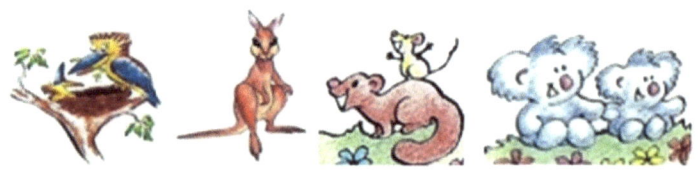

I -'ve cleaned all my mouth

I -'ve cleaned all my mouth

I want a hap -py mouth

I -'ve cleaned all my mouth

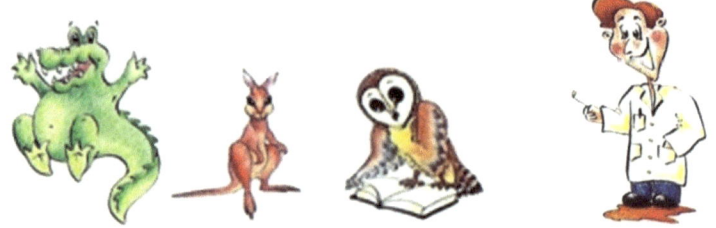

Book 2 of 12:: Your Healthy Whole Mouth.

Learn the Lyrics and Melody of GarGar the Dentist's Song Mouth Painting I will Go

DR Garth Pettit

Then next I rinse and spit

Then next I rinse and spit

I want a mouth wise mouth

Then next I rinse and spit

Now all my mouth is clean

Now all my mouth is clean

I want a heal -thy mouth

Now all my mouth is clean

It's time to paint my mouth

It's time to paint my mouth

I want a hap -py mouth

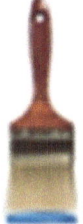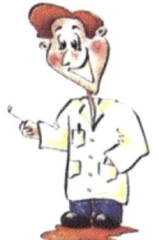

It's time to paint my mouth

Book 2 of 12:: Your Healthy Whole Mouth.

Learn the Lyrics and Melody of GarGar the Dentist's Song Mouth Painting I will Go

DR Garth Pettit

First I paint   the   top   teeth

First I paint   the   top   teeth

I want a mouth wise mouth

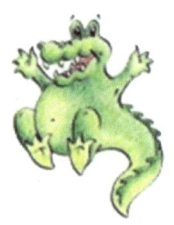 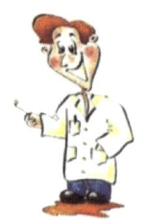

First I paint   the top teeth

Then paint the bot –tom teeth

Then paint the bot –tom teeth

I want a heal -thy mouth

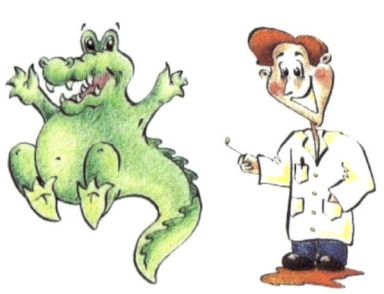

Then paint the bot –tom teeth

Book 2 of 12:: Your Healthy Whole Mouth.

Learn the Lyrics and Melody of GarGar the Dentist's Song Mouth Painting I will Go

DR Garth Pettit

I paint all my top gums

    I paint all my top gums

      I want a hap -py mouth

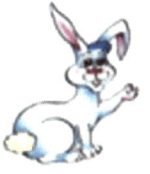

    I paint all my top gums

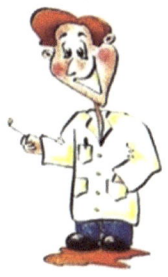

    Then paint all bot –tom gums

    Then paint all bot –tom gums

    I want a mouth wise mouth

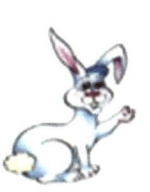 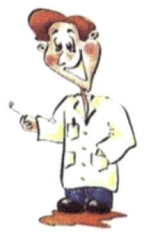

Then paint all bot –tom gums

Book 2 of 12:: Your Healthy Whole Mouth.

Learn the Lyrics and Melody of GarGar the Dentist's Song Mouth Painting I will Go

DR Garth Pettit

I paint all over my tongue

I paint all over my tongue

I want a heal -thy mouth

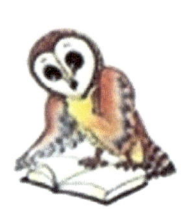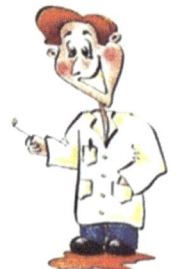

I paint all over my tongue

Paint bub -bles fill my   mouth

Paint bub -bles fill my   mouth

I want a hap -py mouth

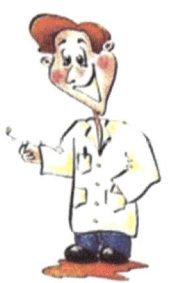

Paint bub -bles fill my   mouth

Book 2 of 12:: Your Healthy Whole Mouth.

Learn the Lyrics and Melody of GarGar the Dentist's Song Mouth Painting I will Go

DR Garth Pettit

This time I do   not   rinse

This time I do   not   rinse

I want a mouth -wise   mouth

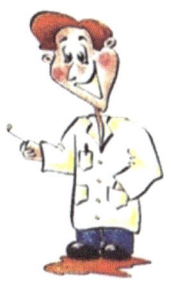

This time I do   not   rinse

I close my lips   and   swish

I close my lips   and   swish

I want a heal   -thy   mouth

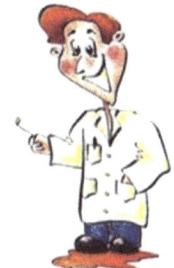

I close my lips and swish

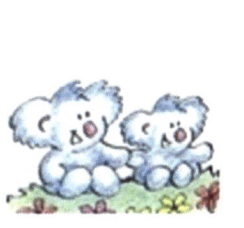

Book 2 of 12:: Your Healthy Whole Mouth.

Learn the Lyrics and Melody of GarGar the Dentist's Song Mouth Painting I will Go

DR Garth Pettit

    I   suck paint   'tween my   teeth

    I   suck paint   'tween my   teeth

    I want a hap -py mouth

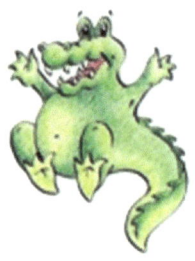

    I   suck paint   'tween my   teeth

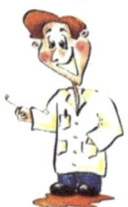

    I   spit out paint   bub –bles

    I   spit out paint   bub -bles

    I want a mouth wise mouth

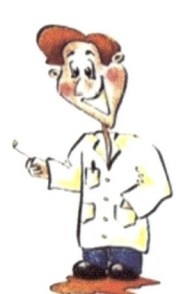

    I   spit out paint   bub -bles

Book 2 of 12:: Your Healthy Whole Mouth.

Learn the Lyrics and Melody of GarGar the Dentist's Song Mouth Painting I will Go

DR Garth Pettit

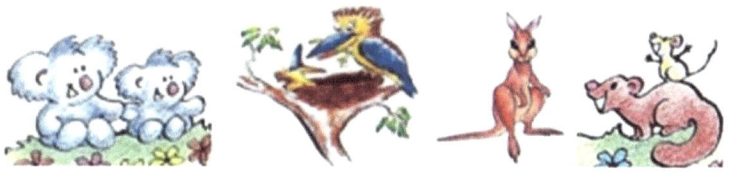

That's how I paint my mouth

That's how I paint my mouth

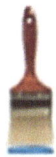

I want a   heal -thy   mouth

That's how I paint my mouth

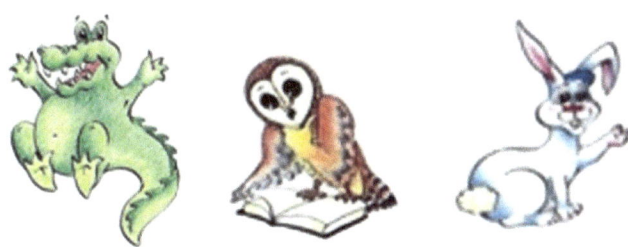

Book 2 of 12:: Your Healthy Whole Mouth.

Learn the Lyrics and Melody of GarGar the Dentist's Song Mouth Painting I will Go

DR Garth Pettit

Might jump o -ver the moon

Might jump o -ver the moon

I want a heal thy Mouth

Might jump o -ver the moon

My mouth's now pro –tec –ted

My mouth's now pro –tec –ted

I have a mouth wise mouth

My mouth's now pro –tec –ted

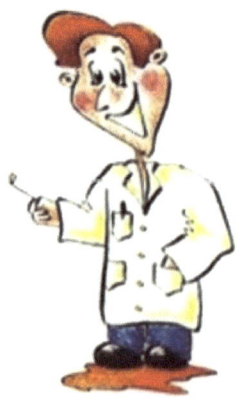

Book 2 of 12:: Your Healthy Whole Mouth.

Learn the Lyrics and Melody of GarGar the Dentist's Song Mouth Painting I will Go

DR Garth Pettit

I will not get bad teeth

I will not get bad teeth

I have a mouth wise mouth

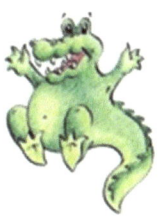

I will not get bad teeth

Bad teeth I now pre -vent

Bad teeth I now pre -vent

I have a mouth wise mouth

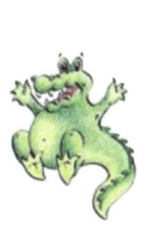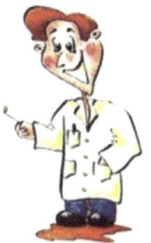

Bad teeth I now pre -vent

Book 2 of 12:: Your Healthy Whole Mouth.

Learn the Lyrics and Melody of GarGar the Dentist's Song Mouth Painting I will Go

DR Garth Pettit

I will not get bad gums

I will not get bad gums

I have a mouth wise mouth

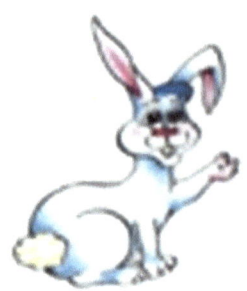

I will not get bad gums

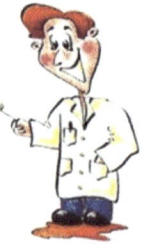

Bad gums I now pre -vent

Bad gums I now pre -vent

I have a mouth wise mouth

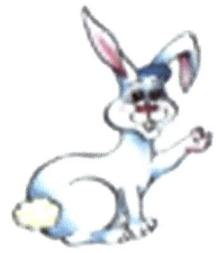

Bad gums I now pre -vent

Book 2 of 12:: Your Healthy Whole Mouth.

Learn the Lyrics and Melody of GarGar the Dentist's Song Mouth Painting I will Go

DR Garth Pettit

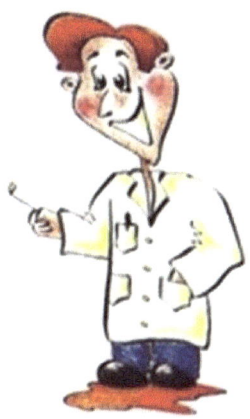

I will not get bad breath

I will not get bad breath

I have a mouth wise mouth

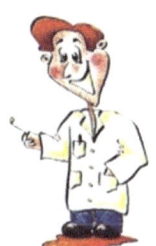

I will not get bad breath

Book 2 of 12:: Your Healthy Whole Mouth.

Learn the Lyrics and Melody of GarGar the Dentist's Song Mouth Painting I will Go

DR Garth Pettit

Bad   breath I now pre -vent

Bad   breath I now pre -vent

I have a mouth wise mouth

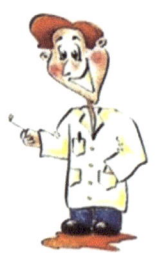

Bad   breath I now pre -vent

I   will   not   have bad   smiles

I   will   not   have bad   smiles

I have a mouth wise mouth

I   will   not   have bad   smiles

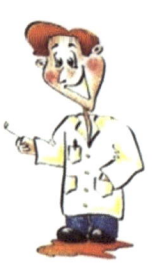

Book 2 of 12:: Your Healthy Whole Mouth.

Learn the Lyrics and Melody of GarGar the Dentist's Song Mouth Painting I will Go

DR Garth Pettit

Bad   smiles I now pre   -vent

      Bad   smiles I now pre   -vent

      I have a mouth wise mouth

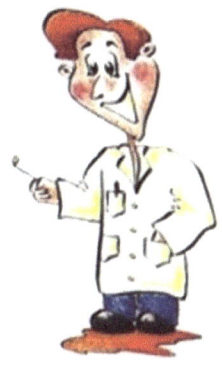

      Bad   smiles I now pre   -vent

      My whole mouth is heal -thy

      My whole mouth is heal -thy

      I have a mouth -wise mouth

      My whole mouth is heal –thy

Book 2 of 12:: Your Healthy Whole Mouth.

Learn the Lyrics and Melody of GarGar the Dentist's Song Mouth Painting I will Go

DR Garth Pettit

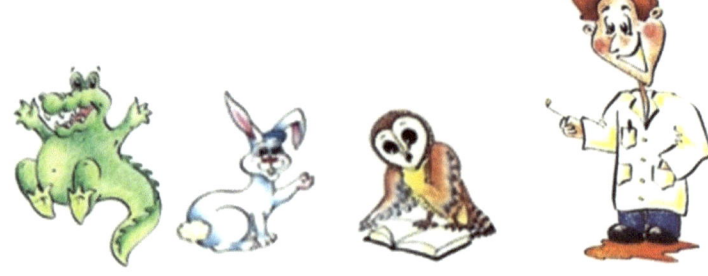

My whole mouth is hap -py

My whole mouth is hap -py

I have a mouth -wise mouth

My whole mouth is hap -py

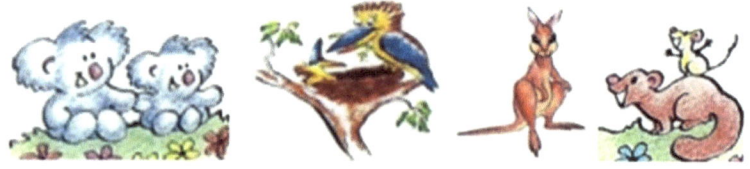

Book 2 of 12:: Your Healthy Whole Mouth.

Learn the Lyrics and Melody of GarGar the Dentist's Song Mouth Painting I will Go

DR Garth Pettit

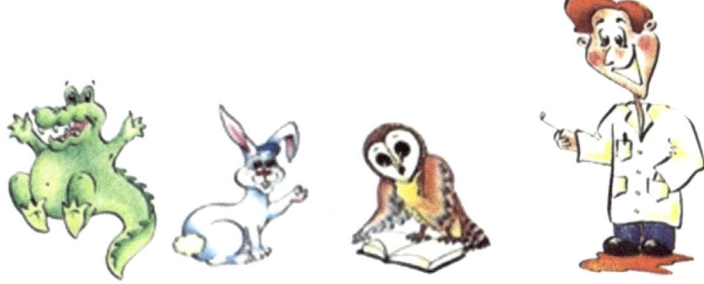

My whole mouth is mouth -wise

My whole mouth is mouth -wise

I have a mouth -wise mouth

My whole mouth is mouth –wise

Book 2 of 12:: Your Healthy Whole Mouth.

Learn the Lyrics and Melody of GarGar the Dentist's Song Mouth Painting I will Go

DR Garth Pettit

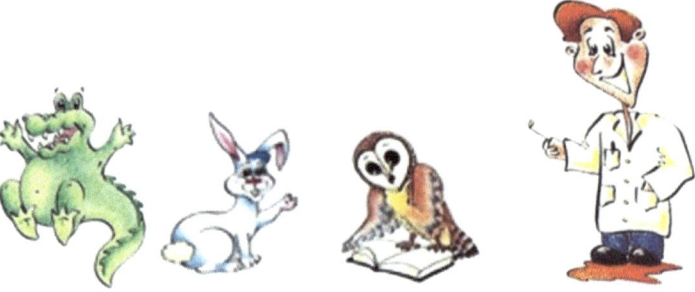

I smile and smile and smile

I smile and smile and smile

I have a mouth wise mouth

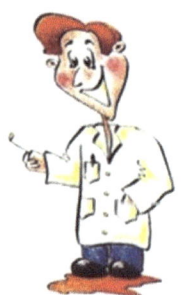

I smile and smile and smile

Book 2 of 12:: Your Healthy Whole Mouth.

Learn the Lyrics and Melody of GarGar the Dentist's Song Mouth Painting I will Go

DR Garth Pettit

I   laugh and laugh and laugh

I laugh and laugh and laugh

I have a mouth wise mouth

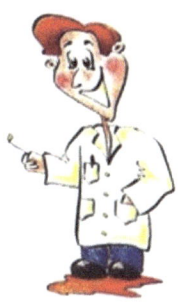

I   laugh and laugh and laugh

The den -tist loves my mouth

The den -tist loves my mouth

I have a mouth wise mouth

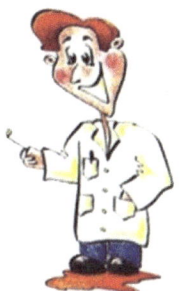

The den -tist loves my mouth

Book 2 of 12:: Your Healthy Whole Mouth.

Learn the Lyrics and Melody of GarGar the Dentist's Song Mouth Painting I will Go

DR Garth Pettit

Gar -Gar ad -ores my mouth

Gar -Gar ad -ores my mouth

I have a mouth wise mouth

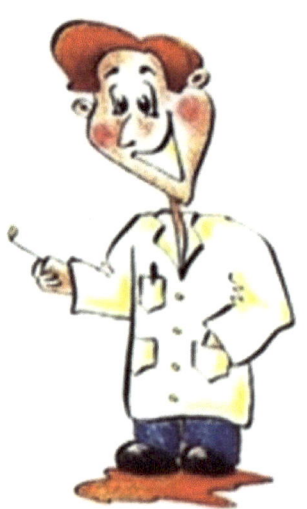

Gar -Gar ad -ores my mouth

Book 2 of 12:: Your Healthy Whole Mouth.

Learn the Lyrics and Melody of GarGar the Dentist's Song Mouth Painting I will Go

DR Garth Pettit

My whole mouth is heal -thy

My whole mouth is hap -py

I have a mouth -wise mouth

Heal –thy hap –py mouth –wise

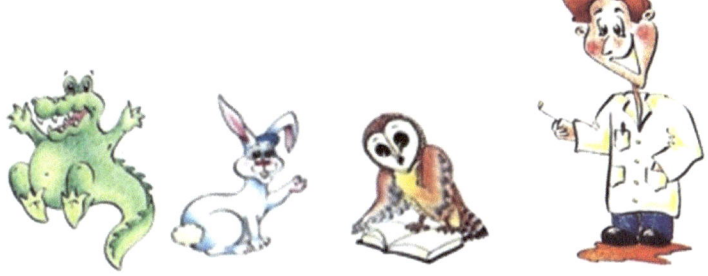

Book 2 of 12:: Your Healthy Whole Mouth.

Learn the Lyrics and Melody of GarGar the Dentist's Song Mouth Painting I will Go

DR Garth Pettit

It's   time for us to go
It's   time for us to go
We have mouth wise mouths
It's   time for us to go

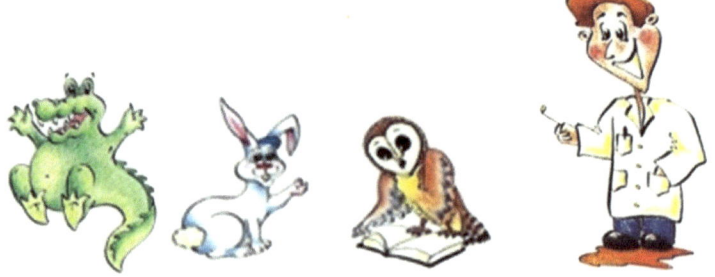

Book 2 of 12:: Your Healthy Whole Mouth.

Learn the Lyrics and Melody of GarGar the Dentist's Song Mouth Painting I will Go

DR Garth Pettit

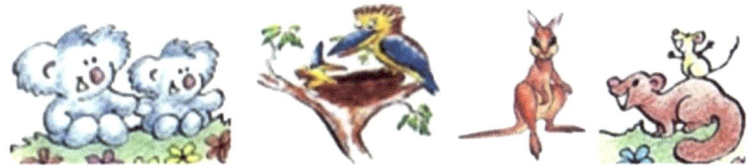

Good -bye good -bye good –bye

Good -bye good -bye good –bye

We all have mouthwise mouths

Good -bye good -bye good –bye

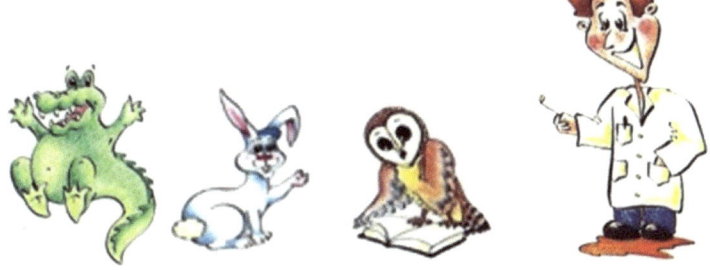

Book 2 of 12:: Your Healthy Whole Mouth.

Learn the Lyrics and Melody of GarGar the Dentist's Song Mouth Painting I will Go

DR Garth Pettit

Chapter 6

Author's eBooks

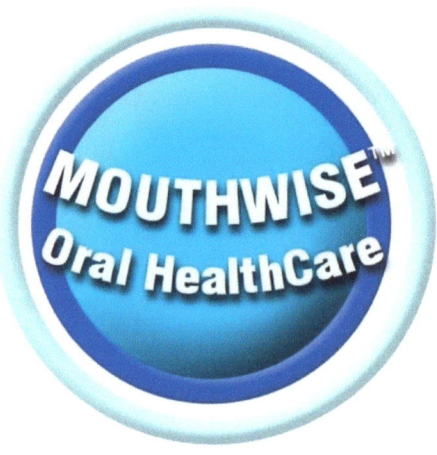

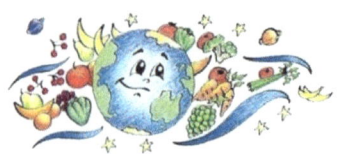

Book 2 of 12:: Your Healthy Whole Mouth.

Learn the Lyrics and Melody of GarGar the Dentist's Song Mouth Painting I will Go

DR Garth Pettit

Of the Author's 86 books available from Amazon two are 2 Paperbacks and the remainder are eBooks. The foreign language eBooks are yet be translated.

Check them here:

https://www.amazon.com/-/e/B007X8KFIY

The eBooks in this series are each

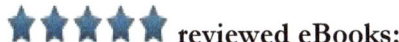 reviewed eBooks:

Please note: eBooks titled *How Do I Look After My Kids* Teeth were, in 2013, re-titled *Teaching Oral Disease Prevention.*

Teaching Oral Disease Prevention. 1 of 12

Teaching Oral Disease Prevention. 2 of 12

Teaching Oral Disease Prevention. 3 of 12

Teaching Oral Disease Prevention. 4 of 12

Teaching Oral Disease Prevention. 5 of 12

Teaching Oral Disease Prevention. 6 of 12

Teaching Oral Disease Prevention. 7 of 12

Teaching Oral Disease Prevention. 8 of 12

Book 2 of 12:: Your Healthy Whole Mouth.

Learn the Lyrics and Melody of GarGar the Dentist's Song Mouth Painting I will Go

DR Garth Pettit

Teaching Oral Disease Prevention. 9 of 12

Teaching Oral Disease Prevention. 10 of 12

Teaching Oral Disease Prevention. 11 of 12

Teaching Oral Disease Prevention. 12 of 12

The following title, combining all 12 books above, is

Twice ★★★★★ reviewed:

Teaching Oral Disease Prevention 1 thru 12

All of the above eBooks are highly recommended to parents, teachers and schools because they are interactive and numerous graphics are available for downloading for children to keep in their "My GarGar The Dentist Activity Album".

<u>Also available by the author are:</u>

Mothers Teach Foetus All About A Smile. Recommended for mothers during or soon after a pregnancy and then very useful up until toddler age.

GarGar The Dentist Toddlers Activity Books. Book a and *GarGar The Dentist Toddlers Activity Books. Book b*

with many more in this series ending with *Book z*.

Book 2 of 12:: Your Healthy Whole Mouth.

Learn the Lyrics and Melody of GarGar the Dentist's Song Mouth Painting I will Go

DR Garth Pettit

List of Proposed Videos

Video 1. STOP Brushing Your Teeth GO Paint Your Mouth. PUBLISHED

Video 2. Learning Oral Disease Prevention. 1 of 12. PUBLISHED

Video 3. Learning Oral Disease Prevention. 2 of 12. PUBLISHED

Video 4. Learning Oral Disease Prevention. 3 of 12. PUBLISHED

Still to be published are:

Video 5. Learning Oral Disease Prevention. 4 of 12

Video 6. Learning Oral Disease Prevention. 5 of 12

Video 7. Learning Oral Disease Prevention. 6 of 12

Video 8. Learning Oral Disease Prevention. 7 of 12

Video 9. Learning Oral Disease Prevention. 8 of 12

Video 10. Learning Oral Disease Prevention. 9 of 12

Video 11. Learning Oral Disease Prevention. 10 of 12

Video 12. Learning Oral Disease Prevention. 11 of 12

Video 13. Learning Oral Disease Prevention 12. of 12

Book 2 of 12:: Your Healthy Whole Mouth.

Learn the Lyrics and Melody of GarGar the Dentist's Song Mouth Painting I will Go

DR Garth Pettit

Video 14. Mothers Teach Fetus All About a Smile

Video a. GarGar The Dentist & His SmileShine Gang with Toddlers

Video b. GarGar The Dentist & His SmileShine Gang with Toddlers

This video series is intended to continue with Video c and to end with Video Z

Book 2 of 12:: Your Healthy Whole Mouth.

Learn the Lyrics and Melody of GarGar the Dentist's Song Mouth Painting I will Go

DR Garth Pettit

Chapter 7

Book Reviews, Websites, General Information

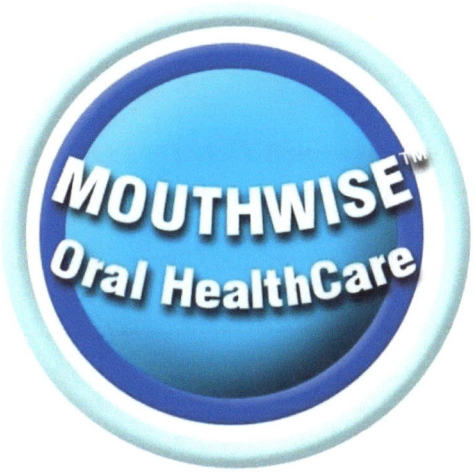

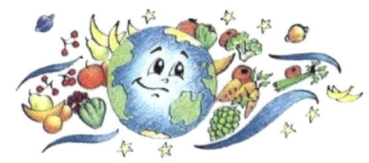

Book 2 of 12:: Your Healthy Whole Mouth.

Learn the Lyrics and Melody of GarGar the Dentist's Song Mouth Painting I will Go

DR Garth Pettit

Firstly, a word about "My GarGar The Dentist Activity Album".

It is an innovative cover graphic for a loose-leaf album in which children can record their eBook drawings, written exercises and numerous free, downloadable graphics that makes teaching using eBooks very simple for parents, teachers and children.

Please note: Books titled *How Do I Look After My Kids* Teeth were, in 2013, re-titled

Teaching Oral Disease Prevention.

Hyperlinks have also been added throughout to download numerous downloadable free graphics such as this "My GarGar The Dentist Activity Album".

This makes teaching with these eBooks a breeze for parents at home and for teachers in schools to educate their children.

Book 2 of 12:: Your Healthy Whole Mouth.

Learn the Lyrics and Melody of GarGar the Dentist's Song Mouth Painting I will Go

DR Garth Pettit

My GarGar The Dentist Activity Album Cover

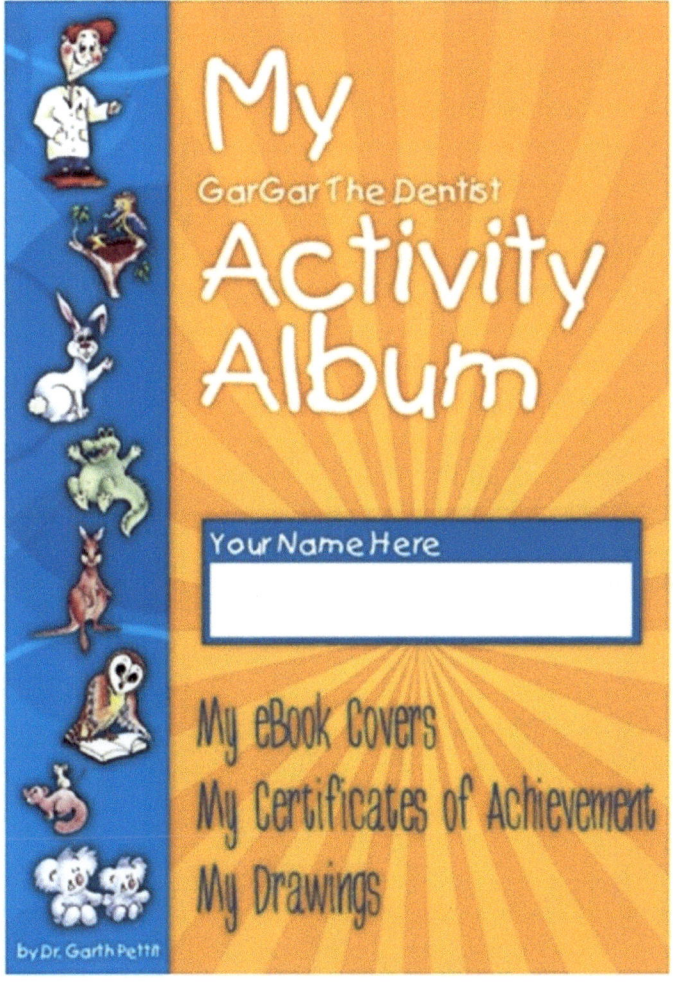

Book 2 of 12:: Your Healthy Whole Mouth.

Learn the Lyrics and Melody of GarGar the Dentist's Song Mouth Painting I will Go

DR Garth Pettit

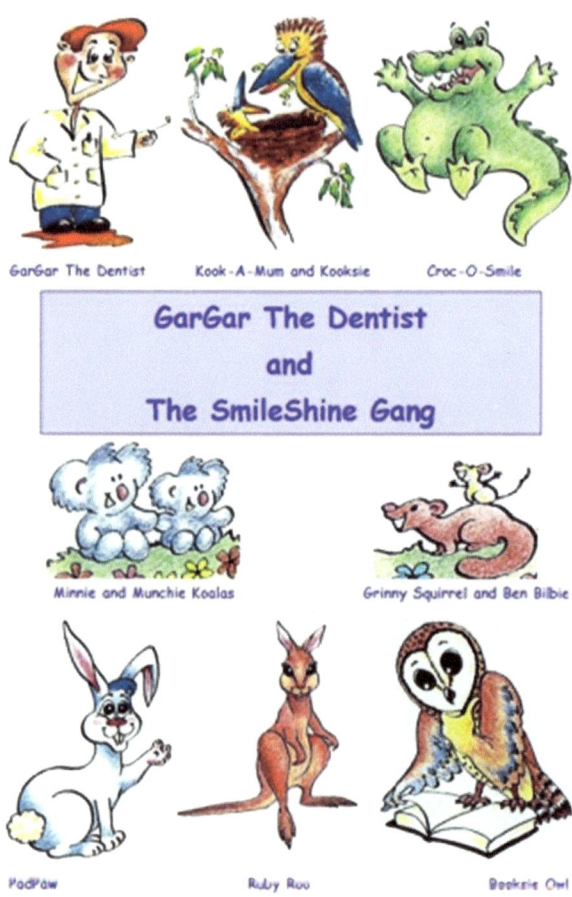

GarGar The Dentist and The SmileShine Gang's

Images and Names

Book 2 of 12:: Your Healthy Whole Mouth.

Learn the Lyrics and Melody of GarGar the Dentist's Song Mouth Painting I will Go

DR Garth Pettit

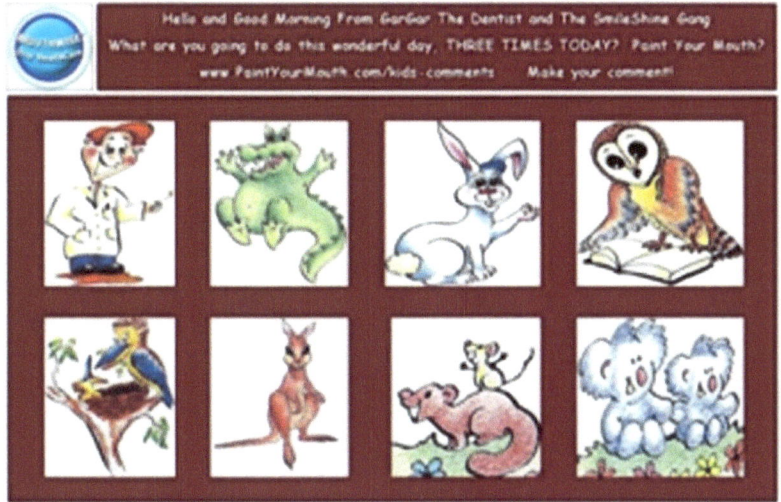

My GarGar The Dentist Bedroom Wall Poster.

Whenever in their bedrooms, several times a day, it will remind them to Paint Your Mouth.

Book 2 of 12:: Your Healthy Whole Mouth.

Learn the Lyrics and Melody of GarGar the Dentist's Song Mouth Painting I will Go

DR Garth Pettit

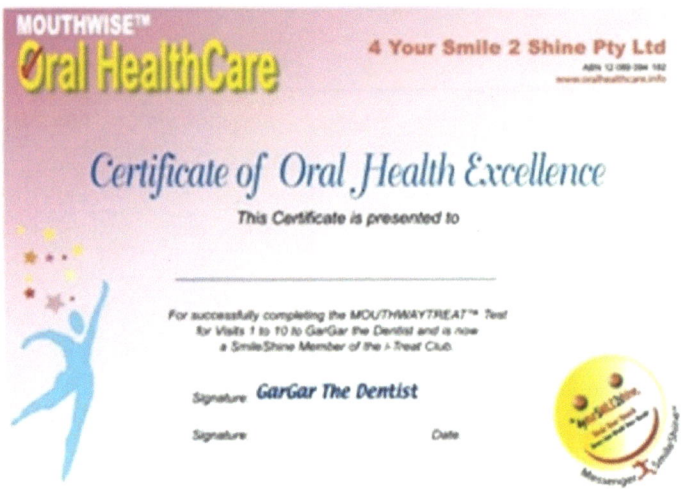

The final of 10 Certificates for their Albums.

When proudly showing off their albums they'll be unwittingly revising!

Book 2 of 12:: Your Healthy Whole Mouth.

Learn the Lyrics and Melody of GarGar the Dentist's Song Mouth Painting I will Go

DR Garth Pettit

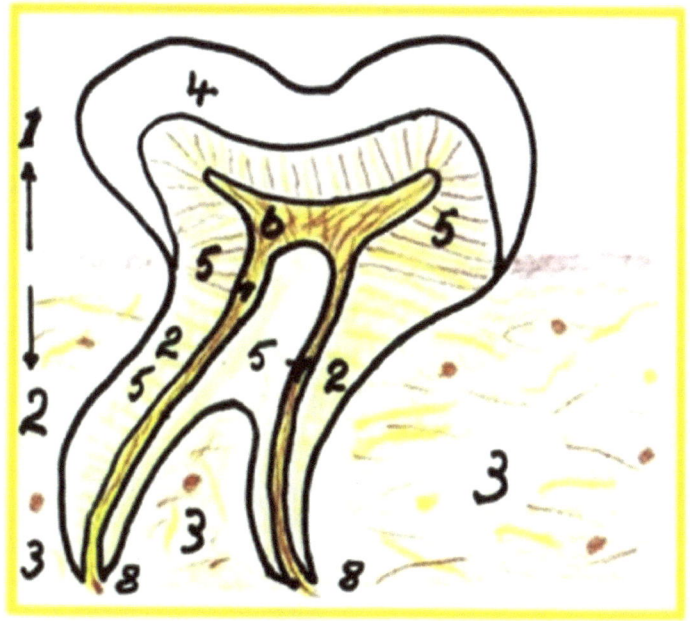

Picture showing parts of a healthy tooth.

Another helpful reminder for their Albums!

Book 2 of 12:: Your Healthy Whole Mouth.

Learn the Lyrics and Melody of GarGar the Dentist's Song Mouth Painting I will Go

DR Garth Pettit

ebook *Mothers Teach Foetus All About A Smile*, a Five Star reviewed book by Diane Donovan, Senior eBook Reviewer, Midwest Book Reviews:

http://www.midwestbookreview.com/mbw/jul_12.htm#donovan

The book series *How Do I Look After My Kids Teeth* 1 of 12, 2 of 12, etc. up to 12 of 12 are each Five Star reviewed books by Diane Donovan, Senior eBook Reviewer, Midwest Book Reviews.

http://www.midwestbookreview.com/mbw/apr_12.htm#donovan

The title How *Do I Look After My Kids Teeth? 1 thru 12* is also a Five Star reviewed book by Diane Donovan, Senior eBook Reviewer, Midwest Book Reviews:

http://www.midwestbookreview.com/mbw/apr_12.htm#donovan

The title How Do I Look After My Kids Teeth? 1 thru 12 has also received a second Five Star review by Cindy Wolfe Boynton, Foreword Clarion Reviews:

https://www.forewordreviews.com/reviews/how-do-i-look-after-my-kids-teeth-1-to-12/

This review follows:

Book 2 of 12:: Your Healthy Whole Mouth.

Learn the Lyrics and Melody of GarGar the Dentist's Song Mouth Painting I will Go

DR Garth Pettit

8 June 2012

ForeWord Clarion

Review: 5 Stars   HEALTH

How Do I Look After My Kids Teeth? 1 thru 12

Dr. Garth Pettit 4 Your Smile 2 Shine Pty. Ltd

978-1-920712-16-7   Five Stars (out of Five)

Retired Australian dentist Garth Pettit, beloved and known to children throughout the world as "GarGar the Dentist," has combined his twelve short *How How Do I Look After My Kids Teeth?* e-books into one comprehensive collection that both children and adults will enjoy and learn from.

Available as an Amazon Kindle e-book, *How Do I Look After My Kids Teeth? 1 thru 12* succinctly illustrates through words and pictures Pettit's "Paint Your Mouth" approach to oral hygiene which, the author explains, kids find much more appealing than being told to "brush [their] teeth."

Adding to the fun is the fact that the book is narrated by Pettit's alter ego, the smiling, animated GarGar the Dentist. Along for the ride is a menagerie of kid-friendly helpers like Booksie Owl, Croc-O-Smile, Grinny Squirrel, and Pad Paw the rabbit who, as members of the SmileShine Gang, offer oral health tips and reminders.

Original songs such as "Mouth Painting I Will Go" sung to the tune of the familiar children's song "A-Hunting We Will Go," also effectively and cleverly disguise learning, as do the Treat Stamps kids can earn for correctly answering questions.

Book 2 of 12:: Your Healthy Whole Mouth.

Learn the Lyrics and Melody of GarGar the Dentist's Song Mouth Painting I will Go

The book also includes drawings, quizzes, and other activities the SmileShine Gang encourages families to do together.

Skilfully woven into these games is the comprehensive healthcare information every young person—and adult—needs to prevent oral problems like tooth decay, gum disease, bad breath, and stained teeth.

Among other topics, readers learn within the book's twelve chapters: the best food and drink options oral for better health; the types of bacteria that form in the mouth; what plaque is and how it forms; what causes bad breath and tooth decay; and the daily steps to the best oral hygiene.

Pettit states that he wrote the twelve *How Do I Look After My Kids Teeth?* e-books to reinforce the lessons kids were hopefully already receiving from their own dentists, schools, and parents. He also wanted to make good oral care something kids would want to do, while understanding why they need to do it.

Without a doubt, Pettit took the right approach. In addition to being written in a kid-friendly tone and including effective graphics, chapters are broken into short, readable sections that can be consumed all at once or bitten into one small chunk at a time.

Sophisticated dental and medical information is presented in a simple, straightforward manner.

At the end of each chapter, both parent and child can show off what they have learned with a printable

Book 2 of 12:: Your Healthy Whole Mouth.

Learn the Lyrics and Melody of GarGar the Dentist's Song Mouth Painting I will Go

DR Garth Pettit

"4 Your Smile to Shine" certificate of achievement

from GarGar the Dentist that will look great on any refrigerator door.

How Do I Look After My Kids Teeth? 1 thru 12 is a well-written, effective, and valuable learning tool for adults and children alike.

Cindy Wolfe Boynton

https://www.forewordreviews.com/reviews/how-do-i-look-after-my-kids-teeth-1-to-12

Since this book was awarded two Five Star Reviews

and a Foreword Clarion Gold Star it has been greatly enhanced and retitled:

Teaching Oral Disease Prevention. 1 thru 12.

Summary of Reviews by D. Donovan

for all thirteen 5 Star Reviews of *How Do I Look After My Kids Teeth?* eBooks

Please note: This eBook has been re-titled and re-published in November 2013 with numerous enhancements under the title:

"*Teaching Oral Disease Prevention. 1 thru 12*".

Book 2 of 12:: Your Healthy Whole Mouth.

Learn the Lyrics and Melody of GarGar the Dentist's Song Mouth Painting I will Go

DR Garth Pettit

A summary of 5 star reviews for the 13 "How Do I Look After My Kids Teeth?" eBooks by D. Donovan, Senior eBook Reviewer, MBR, is below. Links to all reviews are:

http://midwestbookreview.com/mbw/apr_12.htm#donovan/

http://midwestbookreview.com/mbw/jul_12.htm#donovan/

"How, can parents look after their kids' teeth? Plenty of books discuss oral hygiene but most are aimed at adults, and there are very few picture books for young kids - which is where one should ideally begin with early preventative measures."…

"Oral 7 Hygiene: "Paint Your Mouth" is the first book in a series of 12, comes from a dentist who teaches children how to 'paint their mouths', and teaches a preventative program that is much better than just brushing teeth. (In fact, this series shows how brushing teeth often actually leads to poor oral hygiene.)"…

" but their real power lies in the entire lesson plan taken as a whole."…"The step-by-step building blocks of oral health understanding are carefully constructed with the young child in mind, reinforced by activities and quizzes, and provide an entire, unique program unparalleled in scope and nature.

Having the entire lesson plan available in other languages assures its interest to a wide audience around the world, making this entire set a powerful presentation."…"Each
Book 2 of 12:: Your Healthy Whole Mouth.

Learn the Lyrics and Melody of GarGar the Dentist's Song Mouth Painting I will Go

chapter is packed with quizzes, drawing assignments, stamps, certificates of achievement: virtually everything a parent or educator needs to engage a child.

Each chapter also emphasizes the child's power in avoiding tooth decay and bad dental problems."…"Any educator or parent seeking an oral health program directed to the young will find this entire set a winner."

Author's Websites

WorldWide Who's Who, Professional Feature Member 2015 – 2016 http://www.paintyourmouth.com/worldwide-branding-whos-dr-garth-pettit/

WorldWide Who's Who Radio interview: https://goo.gl/syaIsL

My Shopify Address:

https://mouthwise-oral-health-care.myshopify.com/

www.PaintYourMouth.com

www.ExpertClick.com/19-4227

www.prevent-oral-disease-in-children.blogspot.com

Amazon Author Central Account: http://www.amazon.com/-/e/B007X8KFIY

Book 2 of 12:: Your Healthy Whole Mouth.

Learn the Lyrics and Melody of GarGar the Dentist's Song Mouth Painting I will Go

DR Garth Pettit

General Information

Video speech at the "4th Asia Pacific Dental Congress & Expo, Brisbane, Qld. Australia, 27-28-29 July, 2015. Go to: https:www.youtube.com/user/thevideodentist

Video Speech at the 18th Asia Pacific Dental and Oral Care Conference, November 21-23, Melbourne, Australia where Dr. Garth Pettit was Day I Chairperson and Keynote Speaker.

WorldWide Who's Who, Professional Feature Member 2015 – 2016 http://www.paintyourmouth.com/worldwide-branding-whos-dr-garth-pettit/

WorldWide Branding Radio interview: https://goo.gl/syaIsL

FaceBook: www.FACEBOOK.com   **GarthPettit**
Garth.Pettit@Facebook.com

LinkedIn: Dr Garth Pettit

Twitter: Garth Pettit (GarGarDentist)

Google+: Garth D. Pettit

YouTube Channel: TheVideoDentist1

www.Instagram.com **drgarthpettit**

Book 2 of 12:: Your Healthy Whole Mouth.

Learn the Lyrics and Melody of GarGar the Dentist's Song Mouth Painting I will Go

DR Garth Pettit

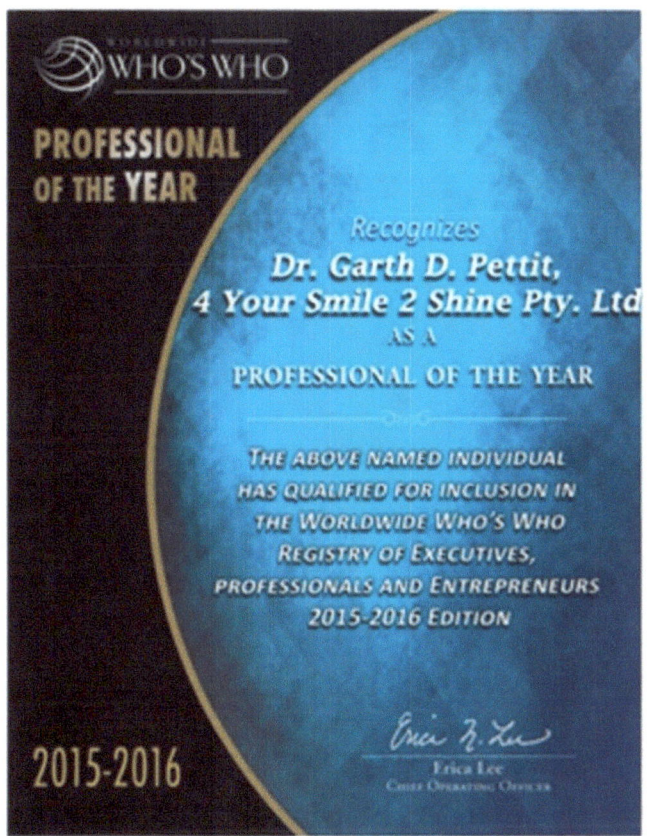

DR Garth D. Pettit,

World Wide Who's Who Professional of The Year

And Chosen Feature Member 2015 – 2016

Book 2 of 12:: Your Healthy Whole Mouth.

Learn the Lyrics and Melody of GarGar the Dentist's Song Mouth Painting I will Go

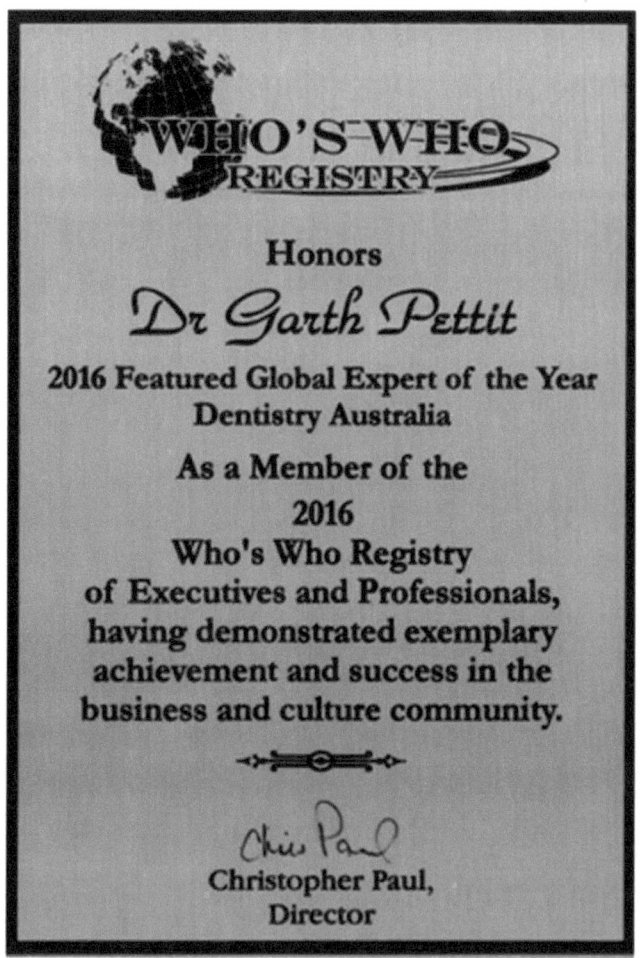

DR Garth Pettit 2016 Featured Global Expert of the Year

Dentistry Australia. Who's Who Registry of the Year

Executives and Professionals

Book 2 of 12:: Your Healthy Whole Mouth.

Learn the Lyrics and Melody of GarGar the Dentist's Song Mouth Painting I will Go

DR Garth Pettit

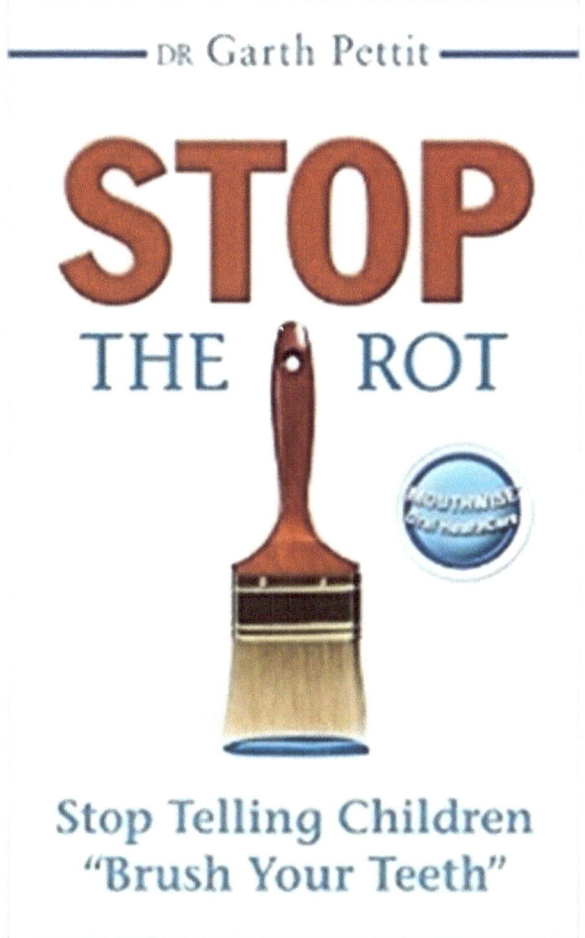

This eBook was Published in 2009 not long before

the author retired from his research because of his wife's ill-health.

Book 2 of 12:: Your Healthy Whole Mouth.

Learn the Lyrics and Melody of GarGar the Dentist's Song Mouth Painting I will Go

DR Garth Pettit

What readers say about "Stop The Rot! Stop Telling Children Brush Your Teeth"...

"As a semi retired itinerant Dentist for the last two years I have worked in many practices in four States. I am yet to find a practice which educates people in the correct use of the so called "tooth" brush. A private dentist would have to charge about $150 to give the full story on how to use this brush - most people wouldn't pay it so they don't 'get' it. This book has it all. Read it. Spread the Word - teach yourself, your kids and your parents"

Richard Conn BDSc

"Reading this outstanding book taught me how to 'treat my whole mouth' which I should have done since I received my first toothbrush. It teaches you so many lessons that everyone should learn. Dr Garth Pettit showed me in person how to do this and reading this book is even better!!

QLD Griffith University Student, Thea J. de Leon

"I am the mother of two children aged 11 and 14 years. When I started reading this book, initially I was horrified. Do not tell my children to brush their teeth?

After I read this book I was totally awed. Wow this book is amazing. It made me realize that go brush your teeth doesn't mean anything. Education is the key. This book makes you open your eyes and realize that there is more to oral health care. I hope now after reading this book I can now educate my children and then they can educate their children. I now know that oral health care is more than just brushing your teeth. This book is fantastic and a wonderful insight into looking after my teeth and my children's teeth and my grand children's teeth."

**Lisa Dawes,
Mother of 2 children.**

HEALTH & FITNESS
Oral Health
ISBN 978-1-60037-542-2

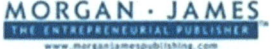
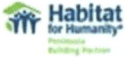

Learn the Lyrics and Melody of GarGar the Dentist's Song Mouth Painting I will Go

DR Garth Pettit

My Dental Patient Testimonials:

Judy Le Cornu, ex-dental assistant and visitor to The Northern Territory, attended for emergency dental treatment on 24 May 2010.

I also gave Judy my oral hygiene instructions "Paint Your Mouth". Here are two emails from Judy.

21 June 2010: "I have accessed your website and am applying your advice regarding cleaning my whole mouth and leaving the toothpaste in my mouth after the second application.

I would like to report to you that the almost total absence of plaque in my mouth is nothing short of amazing.

I have struggled with this all of my life.

I have passed on your advice and website to others and I thank you for taking the time to talk to me about this."

Regards, Judy Le Cornu.

27 June 2010

"My local dentist is an advocate of your oral hygiene methods and after discussing it with her last week she said she will be changing her advice slightly.

Up until now she has been telling her patients to clean the whole mouth but in future will also advise a second brushing and retaining the ingredients of tooth paste. She also said it makes sense so I am spreading the word."

Regards, Judy Le Cornu.

Book 2 of 12:: Your Healthy Whole Mouth.

Learn the Lyrics and Melody of GarGar the Dentist's Song Mouth Painting I will Go

DR Garth Pettit

I do hope you will enjoy my song for many years to come.

May I wish You Happy Total Mouth Health.

Dr Garth Pettit

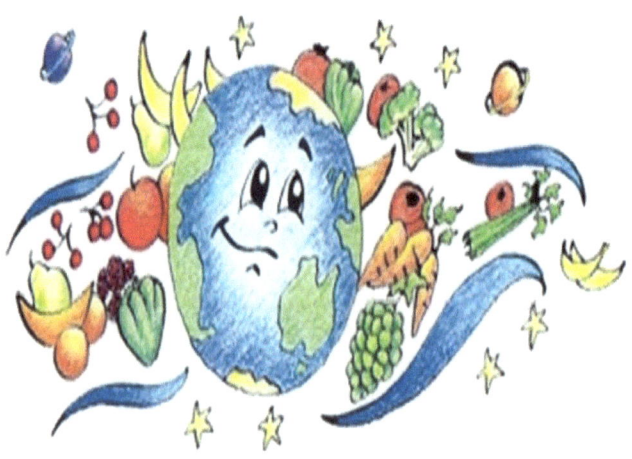

Book 2 of 12:: Your Healthy Whole Mouth.

Learn the Lyrics and Melody of GarGar the Dentist's Song Mouth Painting I will Go

DR Garth Pettit

Book 2 of 12:: Your Healthy Whole Mouth.

Learn the Lyrics and Melody of GarGar the Dentist's Song Mouth Painting I will Go

DR Garth Pettit

Book 2 of 12:: Your Healthy Whole Mouth.

Learn the Lyrics and Melody of GarGar the Dentist's Song Mouth Painting I will Go

DR Garth Pettit

Book 2 of 12:: Your Healthy Whole Mouth.

Learn the Lyrics and Melody of GarGar the Dentist's Song Mouth Painting I will Go

DR Garth Pettit

Book 2 of 12:: Your Healthy Whole Mouth.

Learn the Lyrics and Melody of GarGar the Dentist's Song Mouth Painting I will Go

DR Garth Pettit

Book 2 of 12:: Your Healthy Whole Mouth.

Learn the Lyrics and Melody of GarGar the Dentist's Song Mouth Painting I will Go

DR Garth Pettit

Book 2 of 12:: Your Healthy Whole Mouth.

Learn the Lyrics and Melody of GarGar the Dentist's Song Mouth Painting I will Go

DR Garth Pettit

Book 2 of 12:: Your Healthy Whole Mouth.

Learn the Lyrics and Melody of GarGar the Dentist's Song Mouth Painting I will Go

www.ingramcontent.com/pod-product-compliance
Lightning Source LLC
Chambersburg PA
CBHW040226220526
45473CB00001B/132